MW01116313

# CIALIS USAGE GUIDE FOR MEN

*Men's Long-Lasting Erection Pills: Quick-acting, Stay and Get Rock Hard, Unadulterated Mind-Blowing Climax*

Dr. Abigail Garland

# Copyright @2024

This content of this book should only be used for general educational and informative purposes. It should not be used in place of an expert medical advice, diagnosis or care. In fact, you should always consult your health care provider if you have any questions about a medical issue

# Table of Contents

# Chapter One

## Introduction

If you're trying to find a solution for erectile dysfunction, this book can be beneficial.

Medical professionals have determined that the inability to obtain or maintain an erection is significant, and Cialis (tadalafil) is one of the drugs that is most commonly prescribed to treat it.

Male sexual performance is impacted by erectile dysfunction, which is treated with tadalafil. This medication is categorized as a phosphodiesterase 5 (PDE5) inhibitor, a class of medications.

Phosphodiesterase type-5 is prematurely inhibited by these medicines. One place where this enzyme is active is the penis.

The term "erectile dysfunction" refers to a man's incapacity to maintain an erection following six thrilling sexual experiences.

Although a man's biology naturally increases blood flow to his penis in response to sexual stimulation, tadalafil lengthens an erection by regulating the enzyme.

Tadalafil will not produce an erection in the absence of a physical stimulus to the penis, such as that which happens during sexual activity.

Men who exhibit the warning signs and symptoms of benign prostatic hyperplasia (BPH) can also be treated with tadalafil. BPH is mostly caused by an enlarged condition. Males with benign prosthetic hyperplasia (BPH) typically have reduced urine flow at first, difficulty voiding, and midnight urination.

Tadalafil may lessen the severity of symptoms and maybe eliminate the need for prostate surgery. The symptoms of BPH and erectile dysfunction are also treated with this medication.

Men and women are taken tadalafil to alleviate the symptoms of pulmonary arterial hypertension and enhance their level of exercise.

This hypertension affects the primary blood vessel from the ventricle on the right side of the heart. In order to pump blood into the lungs, the right ventricle has to work harder when the tiny blood capillaries in the lungs become less permeable.

Tadalafil relaxes blood arteries by acting on the PDE5 enzyme in the lungs. As a result, the heart will work harder while pumping more blood to the lungs.

The US Food and Drug Administration (USFDA) authorized tadalafil in 2003 as a remedy for erectile dysfunction.

Low libido or erectile dysfunction are not improved by Cialis or other PDE5 inhibitors. Nevertheless, the use of medications to help achieve and sustain an erection requires both psychological and physical application.

Nitric oxide (NO) is released when the parasympathetic nervous system is triggered, which occurs during sexual desire. Elevated NO levels lead to increased cyclic GMP production.

More blood can enter the penis since Cialis for ED relaxes the arteries that supply it. Essien reduces the signs and symptoms of BPH and makes it easier to urinate since it relaxes the muscles in the bladder. Only those with a prescription can buy Cialis.

# Chapter Two

# Taking Cialis

The penis swells with blood during a penile erection. This is so because the veins supplying the penis allow for unhindered blood flow. As a result, the blood vessels originating from the penis degenerate. A blood clot forms in the penis during an erection.

Cialis also inhibits the effects of a prescription medication that the body frequently transports into the penis during sexual activity as part of its mode of action. As a result, the penis is now within the reach of the stream design. Erections are usually caused by a rise in blood flow to particular inner penile regions.

Nitric oxide finally makes its way to the penis, where it enhances a man's attractiveness. cGMP and nitric oxide regulate the blood arteries that supply and drain the penile region. PDE5 is an alternate atom that outperforms cGMP. The veins return to their resting position after the erection has ended.

When using Cialis, PDE5 is unable to perform better than cGMP. This may lead to an erection that lasts longer.

Given that PDE5 is present in the muscles around the lungs' dividing veins, this pharmacological approach may aid in the treatment of pneumonic hypertension.

# Chapter Three

## Using Cialis

Cialis is sold as 5–20 mg yellow, film-coated, almond-shaped pills. Cialis is a prescription drug used to treat erectile dysfunction (ED), or male sexual dysfunction.

When combined with sexual stimulation, tadalafil helps a man get and sustain an erection by increasing blood flow to the penis.

This medicine does not result in erections when administered in the absence of any sexual stimulation. When the drug is triggered, the proper conditions must be met for it to start working.

BPH symptoms include weak streams, frequent impulses to urinate, and difficulty initiating the flow of urine during urination. Tadalafil is another medication used to treat these symptoms. It is commonly recognized that tadalafil relaxes the bladder's and prostate's smooth muscles.

Furthermore, it does not treat communicable infections including syphilis, gonorrhea, hepatitis B, or HIV. For more information, speak with your doctor or pharmacist. Before starting to take tadalafil, read the Patient Information Leaflet that your doctor provided you. After that, read it again before getting a refill. If you have any concerns, consult a medical professional, such as your primary care physician.

As directed by your doctor, take this medication orally, either with or without food. It is advised to just take tadalafil once day. The estimate will vary depending on your drug use history, treatment response, and the severity of your ailment.

See your primary care physician or a pharmacist to learn additional details about the medications you are taking. Prescription and over-the-counter medications as well as common goods are covered.

For Cialis, there are two dosage options. Your doctor can advise you on the optimal Cialis dosage. Make sure you carefully follow your doctor's instructions because the method you take your medication changes the dosage.

A starting dose of 10 mg should be administered for the first technique 30 minutes prior to engaging in sexual activity. Tadalafil use may have an impact on sexual function for up to 36 hours.

A dosage adjustment may then be necessary based on the patient's response. The most extreme approach, in any case, is a single dose of 20 mg. One dosage is permitted every 24 hours.

However, a daily dose of 10–20 mg is not recommended because drug fragments can stay in the bloodstream for up to 24 hours.

If patients choose to engage in dynamic, active behavior (such as sexual engagement), they may take 5 mg twice weekly; however, the dosage may be lowered to 2.5 mg depending on the patient's reaction.

Cialis is a prescription drug for erectile dysfunction that is available to both men and women over the age of 18.

The next step in the treatment of erectile dysfunction is to take Cialis regularly. If you have sex frequently, you can have it whenever you want. To treat the symptoms of BPH, use this drug once daily as directed by your physician. If you're taking finasteride to treat BPH symptoms, speak with your doctor or pharmacist about the appropriate dosage and length of use.

If you use Cialis as directed and have both BPH and erectile dysfunction, take one dosage per day. Sexual activity can occur at irregular intervals.

The medication should be taken daily to treat ED, BPH, or both.

You should set up periodic reminders to help you remember to take your medicine. Make an appointment with your doctor if the situation neither improves nor becomes worse.

# Chapter Four

## Side Effects

Combining tadalafil or Cialis with a nitrate supplement will dramatically reduce your blood pressure, also referred to as hypertension.

If you are taking a nitrate for heart problems or chest discomfort, you should not use Cialis.

Seek immediate medical attention if any of the following signs of real complexity manifest during sexual activity:

- headaches

- Constipation

- back pain

- Muscle soreness and aches

- obstruction of the nose

- Floshing

- lightheadedness

If any of these side effects worsen or continue, please contact your primary care physician or a pharmaceutical expert immediately.

By rising gently from a sitting or sleeping posture, you can lessen the likelihood of experiencing fatigue and confusion.

Remember that this drug has more advantages than disadvantages, which is why your doctor prescribed it to you. Many people who use this drug report very minimal side effects.

If you already have heart problems, having sex can dramatically exacerbate heart strain. In addition to cardiac problems, if you have any of the following symptoms, you should cease having sex right away and consult a physician.

- lightheadedness

- swooning

- ache in the chest

- jaw soreness

- arms hurting.

- emesis

Long-term visual impairment (NAION) is an uncommon consequence of an abrupt loss of vision in one or both eyes.

If this dangerous situation occurs, immediately stop taking tadalafil and seek medical attention. Smoking, high blood pressure, diabetes, high cholesterol, hypertension, several other eye disorders ("crowded disk"), or being older than 50 all somewhat enhance your chance of NAION.

Rarely, a person may experience a sudden loss of hearing, sometimes with ringing in the ears and dizziness. If you have any of these side effects, immediately cease taking Tadalafil and consult a doctor.

If you have an uncomfortable or delayed erection that lasts more than four hours, you should stop taking this medicine as soon as possible and seek medical attention. If you don't, you face the risk of encountering problems once more.

Using this drug seldom results in serious hypersensitivity reactions. Seek emergency medical assistance if you develop a rash, tingling or swelling (especially on the face, tongue, or throat), severe wooziness, or difficulty falling asleep.

The outcomes are by no means comprehensive. See your primary care physician or a pharmaceutical expert if you have any other unpleasant side effects that are not included in this list.

# Chapter Five

# Those who can't take Cialis

If you have any of the following conditions, you can only use Cialis with your doctor's consent and prescription:

1.  infection in the kidneys or liver.

2.  an ulcer within the stomach.

something that keeps people from engaging in sexual activity.

It is possible to obtain several blood pressure readings. Individuals may be affected by hemophilia, leukemia, myeloma, leukopenia, sickle cell anemia, and other blood disorders.

Retinitis pigmentosa is one type of retinitis that affects the eyes.

You suffered from myocardial dead tissue, congestive heart failure, or a stroke during the last three or six months. Peyronie's sickness, for example, modifies the anatomy of the penis. Consider angina, or any heart ailment for that matter.

# Chapter Six

## Precautions

Inform your doctor or pharmacist if you have ever had hypertension or any other sensitivity before starting Cialis. Inactive substances in this product have the potential to cause hypertension and other health problems. For further information, consult a professional or your pharmacist.

Discuss your medical history with your physician or pharmacist, especially if you have ever had any of the following conditions: stroke, angulation, fibrosis/scarring in the penis, liver disease, kidney disease, high or low blood pressure, cardiovascular breakdown, angina, chest pain, or a history of problematic or delayed erections (priapism).

One side effect of tadalafil is dizziness. Drinking alcohol or smoking marijuana can both lead to inebriation. Before operating a vehicle, utilizing any equipment, or performing any other activity that requires availability, hold off until you are certain that you can finish the task safely. It shouldn't be used extensively. Speak with your doctor before using marijuana.

Discuss all of the medications you use, including over-the-counter products, professional prescriptions, and medications suggested by non-specialists, with your doctor or a dental expert prior to surgery.

This medication is not intended for use by women. When pregnant, use it only when absolutely essential. Discuss the benefits and drawbacks of any drug with your doctor before taking it.

Before nursing, find out from your doctor if this medication is excreted in breast milk.

# Chapter Seven

## Interactions

Drug interactions can significantly impair your health or alter the way your prescriptions function. This is by no means an exhaustive list. Enumerate all the products you use, including herbal, prescription, and over-the-counter supplements.

You should discuss this list with a pharmaceutical expert as well as your primary care provider. It is never a good idea to start, stop, or switch drugs without first consulting your primary care physician. One drug that may interact with this one is riciguat.

When tadalafil and nitrates are taken together, blood pressure can drop significantly, increasing the risk of fainting, blackouts, and, in rare cases, heart failure or stroke. If you take nitrates (nitroglycerine, isosorbide), sports medications that contain butyl or amyl nitrite, or some angina therapies, use tadalafil with caution.

If you use an alpha blocker (doxazosin or tamsulosin, for example, to treat BPH or hypertension) and have dizziness or blackouts, your pulse may drop too low.

To reduce the risk of low blood pressure, your primary care physician may adjust the amount of tadalafil you take or switch the alpha blocker you take.

Tadalafil may leave your body in a different way depending on the prescription, which could affect how well it functions. Examples include the macrolide antibiotics erythromycin and clarithromycin, the HIV protease inhibitors ritonavir and fosamprenavir, rifampin, boceprevir and telaprevir for hepatitis C, itraconazole, and ketoconazole.

In case you suffer from pulmonary hypertension or erectile dysfunction, stay away from taking tadalafil or comparable drugs (vardenafil, sildenafil, etc.) while using this medication.

# Chapter Eight

## Overdose

Tadalafil, the main ingredient in Cialis, aids in maintaining powerful erections. Cialis overdoses have been reported, though they can also happen accidentally on occasion. Overuse of this medication may result in symptoms and adverse effects.

If you believe you may have overdosed on a prescription medicine, go to the nearest emergency room or contact your social insurance provider straight once.

**Symptoms of a Cialis Overdose**
You should be aware of the following warning signs of a Cialis overdose:

- Anxiety-related chest discomfort

- Disruption of Heartbeat

- lightheadedness

- Having difficulty staying awake or feeling lightheaded

- emesis

Furthermore, it may increase the likelihood of unfavorable responses like these.

- Headaches

- indigestion

- Cosmetics sterilization

- back discomfort

- A pulled muscle

Nasal congestion is the term used to describe obstruction of the nasal passages.

Particularly sore are the arms and legs.

There can be other symptoms that are not included in this guidebook.

**Treatment for Overdose**
Sedative overdoses need to be notified as soon as possible so that the appropriate care can be provided. The provider of restorative administrations will provide a treatment plan based on the signs and symptoms of medication usage. A specific drug is not used to treat a Cialis overdose. Treatment usually consists of continuing mental exercises.

**Prevention of Overdose**
To avoid an overdose, be aware that Cialis can remain in your bloodstream for up to 72 hours. Usually, patients should take one Cialis pill every day.

The two different dose approaches are as follows: continuous dosage and dosing as needed. For exact dosage recommendations, speak with your doctor or pharmacist.

You should also carefully read the medicine label. If you have any queries concerning the drug or the recommended course of treatment, ask your pharmacist.

Observe the directions on the prescription exactly as prescribed. If the drug isn't working or you need it to start working right now, don't self-medicate. Consider how little effect Cialis has on erections. If you're feeling extremely euphoric, it might help you get an erection.

It is also a good idea to stay away from anything that can interfere with Cialis's processing or mechanism of action. Patients should not, for instance, eat grapefruits or grapefruit juice. Because

Cialis contains grapefruit, the body could not be able to metabolize it, which could result in an overdosage. Take Cialis at least three days after consuming grapefruit juice.

It is not recommended to take Cialis along with other erectile dysfunction drugs like sildenafil (Viagra) or vardenafil (Levitra). Before you answer, make sure you have considered every possibility. Each patient requires specialist care because these diseases only afflict one in eight persons.

### Handling a Missed Dosage

Take your medication as soon as you recall if you tend to forget to take it. If the next dose is soon due, skip the missed one. To make up for lost time, eat your next meal at the same time every day.

# Chapter Nine

## Storage of Cialis

Keep it dry, out of direct sunlight, and at room temperature. Never keep items in the bathroom for storage. Drugs should never be available to children or animals.

Unless otherwise instructed, drugs should not be disposed of or poured into the sink or toilet. When this item expires or is no longer needed, please dispose of it properly.

# The End

Made in the USA
Middletown, DE
06 September 2024